Medicinal and Culinary Herbs
Growing, Drying and Preserving

Table of Contents

Introduction 4

Chapter 1 – Best Medicinal Herbs...5

Chapter 2 – Culinary Herbs and Their Benefits.....................................14

Chapter 3 – Tips to Grow, Dry, and Preserve Medicinal Herbs...........18

Chapter 4 – How to Grow, Dry and Preserve Medicinal Herbs 22

Chapter 5 – Recipes to Use Medicinal and Culinary Herbs 30

Conclusion 33

Introduction

The wisdom of nature is surely unprecedented and it is obvious when we look at various creations all around us. Even the tiniest bud grown in the corner of your garden may have hundreds of utilities unknown to us.

But just as the scientific exploration is getting faster we can now see these hidden benefits with a greater magnifying power. Today hundreds of botanical and herbal species are known which have revolutionary benefits hidden in them. The additional benefit of these botanical species is the absence of any kind of additive or artificial element so no side effect can be claimed.

The term herb refers to any plant which is used as a food, medicine, flavoring agent or perfume. Most of the herbs are used in dried form so just as the knowledge about herbs is increasing there has been a progress in determining various techniques available for drying and preserving techniques applied for gaining benefit from herbs.

This book will unveil a number of different herbs which are the source of medicinal and nutritional benefits. At a household level, these herbs can be grown with no extra effort. In order to attain maximum utility, it is essential to start with the basic knowledge about herbs and their principal uses. □

Chapter 1 – Best Medicinal Herbs

The field of medicine has a long held history as it has traveled across the human civilization. In earlier days the development was not that prominent and raw form of medicine was used.

But even today when science and its related field of medicine have made a lot of progress around seventy percent of pharmaceutical products and twenty percent of drugs are obtained from plants and related botanical species.

A vast number of people around the globe use botanical and herbal in order to attain natural methods of health care. With regard to the medicinal plants and herbs, the place is wider than a curative aspect only.

They often find a tighter and prominent space in the cultural fabric embedded within particular social groups. So you can see Medicinal herbs used as herbal baths, extracts, powders, teas, powders, salves, poultices, or syrups.

Any herbs can have medicinal benefits if there is the presence of some chemical components in the structure of the herb which can provoke a specific response within the human body. The specific dosage and its potency will significantly depend on the specific part of the herb utilized, the particular season on which it is grown, and even upon the specific composition of the soil used to grow the medicinal herb.

The chemical composition of medicinal herbs:

There is some specific composition of medicinal herb which makes them useful for serving the purpose as a curative. For majority of the medical issues herbs are considered useful because of the presence of any of the following chemicals or agents in the herb:

- Terpenes

- Tartaric acids

- Tannins

- Saponins

- Mucilage

- Glycosides

- Flavonoids

- Essential oils

- Coumarins

- Citric acid

- Bitter compounds

- Antibiotics

- Alkaloids

The presence of any of these elements will make sure that that the medicinal properties of herbs are ensured. A lot of medicinal herbs may contain even more than one chemical agent and thus enhancing the curative capabilities of a particular medicine. The mixture of these agents is used in pharmaceutical industry to make up various medicines.

Some commonly used medicinal herbs

Herbs are widely in use for edible purposes as well as for medicinal purposes. Many of them are largely in use but we may not be aware of their medicinal potentials.☐

- **Basil:**

Basil can serve as mild sedative, antiseptic, anti-flatulent, expectorant, and laxative. In the fresh form, just before the bloom of flowers, it is used as a tea to release gastritis, stomach ailments, constipation and various indigestion problems.

Basil has been reported to be capable of treating colds, headaches and colds and throat inflammation. In some cases, it may also help in lowering down the fever. So if you are interested in growing herb at home, basil appears to be a good choice for everyday use.

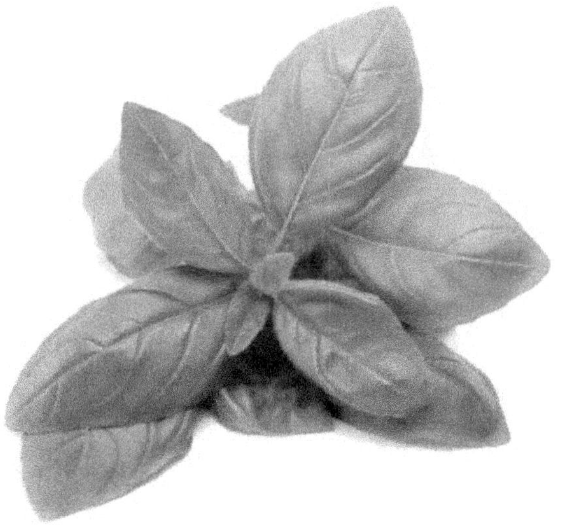

- **Fennel**

This herb has also some great curative properties. It is said to be a diuretic and as the ability to reduce colic. Fennel is given to feeding mothers as its chemical composition induces an increase in milk production.

It also aids in curing digestive disorders, insomnia, coughs, asthma, flatulence, headache, dizziness, catarrh, depression, and inflammation. Moreover, as a household friendly herb, it is used as an insect repellent.

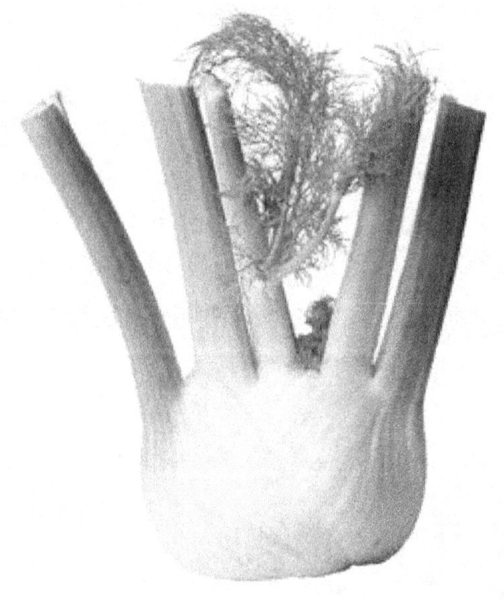

- **Chamomile**

It is best known to have calming properties so it is used to make tea for relaxation and calming nerves.

This herb believed to be curative for the stomach ailment, headaches, colic, flatulence, cold, insomnia and flu symptoms as well as inflammatory issues. It is also helpful to cure hemorrhoids, sore throat, ulcers, acne and a number of eye ailments.

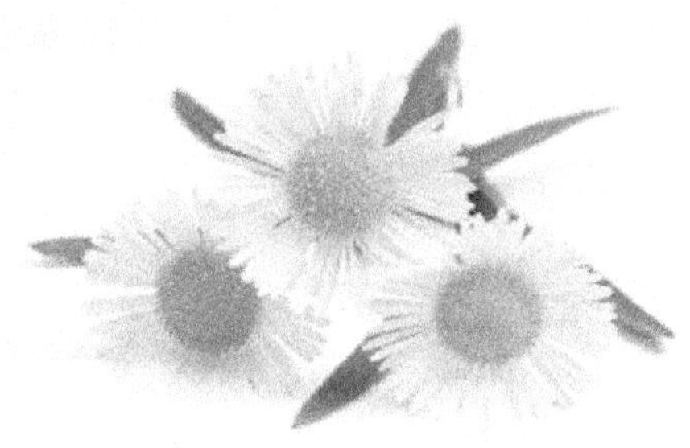

- **Garlic**

Many of you may be using garlic but may not be aware of its medicinal benefits. It has a vast plethora of various curative benefits. It helps in cold, bronchitis, congestion and influenza. It also helps the body to maintain a perfect balance of useful bacteria so that harmful parasite and viruses can be eradicated with a natural system within the body.

Recently medical experts are extending efforts for unveiling the carcinogenic properties of garlic. Some recent studies have also reported the properties of garlic which help in eliminating the risk of strokes and heart attacks.

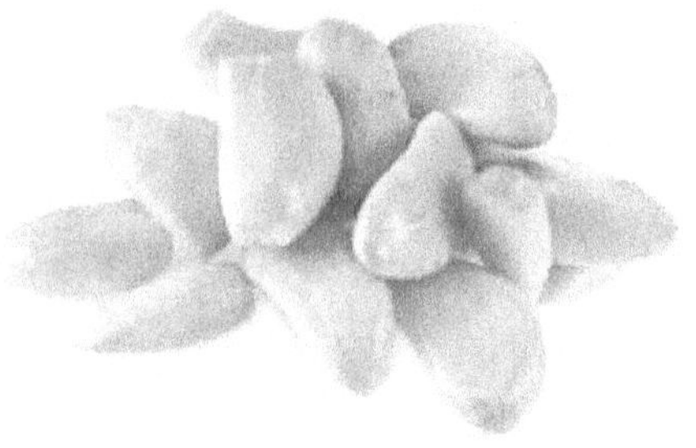

- **Thyme**

It is one of the most ancient herbs which are in use by human civilization. It has an aromatic herb best known for its effective antiseptic properties.

As a medicinal agent, it is used to handle a sore throat, indigestion, coughs, arthritis, and acne. Thyme is also the easiest one to grow, where all you need to do is to put some seedlings of thyme in your garden. Thyme needs sunlight to grow.

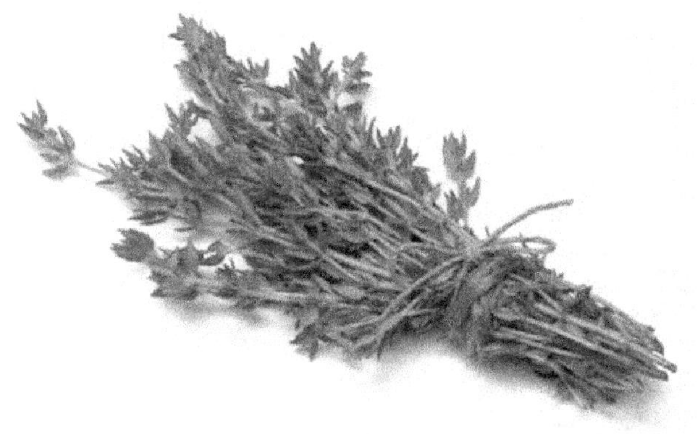

- **Lavender**

This is a beautiful herb with obvious aromatic proteins. Because of its sweet fragrance, it has obvious relaxing and calming properties which are highly beneficial for the human nervous system.

It also helps in reducing pain and entails antiseptic properties. So it is applied to cure bruises and skin cuts. It is a Mediterranean herb, so if you are interested in growing it at your home you need to supply it with the excess of sunlight.

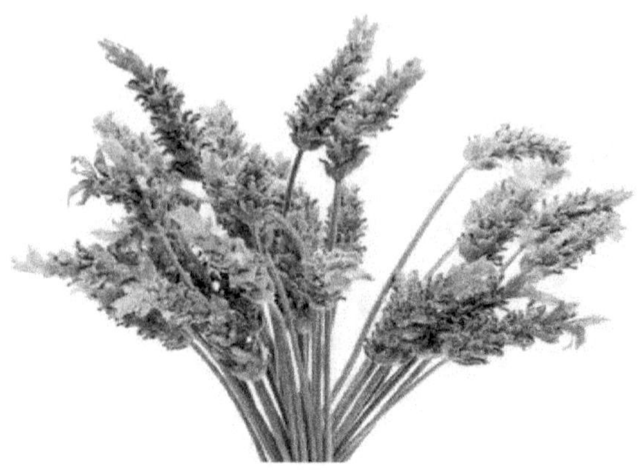

- **Parsley**

Parsley is not only an edible herb used in the variety of meat recipes but is also full of medicinal benefits. It is known to boost the immune system conquer inflammation and prevent diabetes. Parsley is also easy to grow as you will need seed planting. But make sure you have a long container to cater its long roots. It will need a mild exposure to sunlight along with moisture.

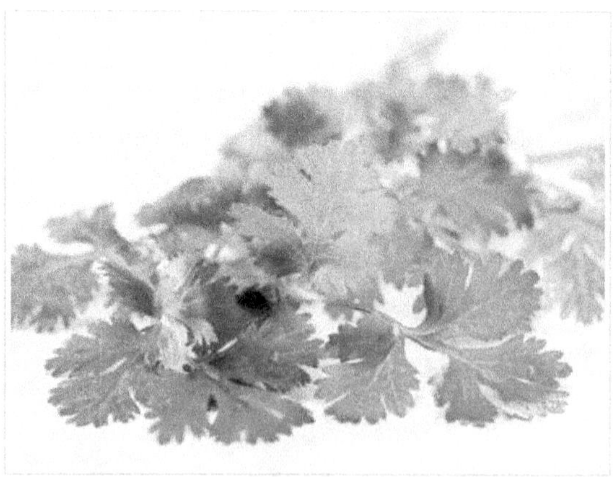

- **Echinacea**

It is a great medicinal herb which is used in a variety of coughs and cold syrups as it helps in lowering down the inflammation of the throat and nasal cavity. It also acts on the human immune system and helps to boost up the working of the immune system.

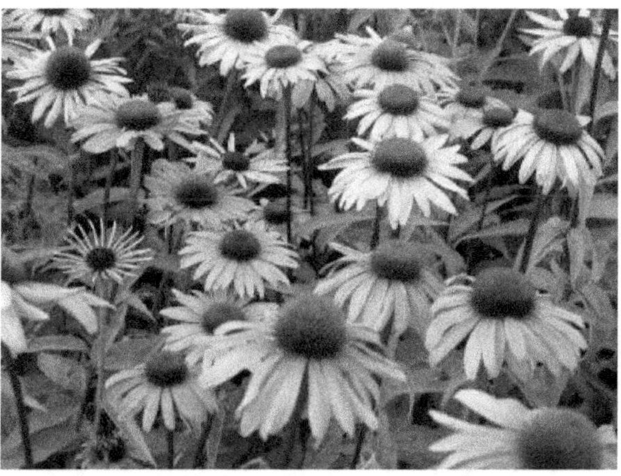

The list for medicinal herbs is quite long and you can learn more about it. But the list mentioned above is the one which is most usable at the household level.

Not only these are helpful for various health issues but these are also useful because of great edible benefits.

Chapter 2 – Culinary Herbs and Their Benefits

Culinary herbs are different from vegetables but fall under the category of herbaceous plants. Being different from spices these are usually used in very small amounts and used to enhance flavor. The basic purpose is not to add rather a substance to food but provides a specific aroma and taste.

Culinary herbs usually exist in two forms. They can either be used in their raw and natural form which is obtained from the garden or kept in store. But when the herb is detached from the main plant the life expectancy of culinary herbs falls and they need to preserve in some proper way.

So these preserved forms of herb fall under the second category in which the herb is said to be dried herb. The concentrated form of herbs has greater aroma and flavor. Culinary herbs are usually obtained from leaves, but flowers root plants or even fruits can be used to obtain these culinary herbs.

Culinary herbs fall into a number of categories and there are around hundreds of herbs available for the use. There are various industrial steps which are grown at various levels in order to obtain large scale growth.

Cinnamon

Cinnamon is one of the useful herbs which enhances the insulin sensitivity and aids largely in burning of calories and fat. It also suppresses stomach ulcers nausea. Cinnamon is also reported to have the anti-inflammatory effects.

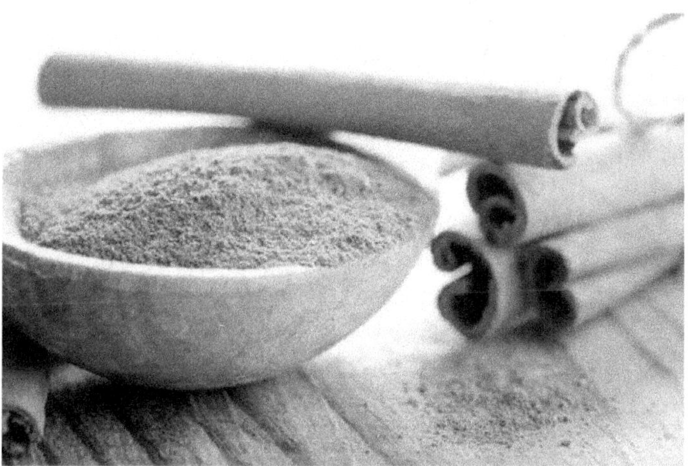

Cinnamon can be taken as raw by stirring into cereal, yogurt, oatmeal, coffee and tea for enhanced flavor. You can also sprinkle it over jelly or peanut butter

Oregano

Oregano is a treasure of antioxidants. Even a tablespoon of oregano is full in antioxidants. Oregano helps largely in loosening mucus, treating respiratory illness and calming indigestion.

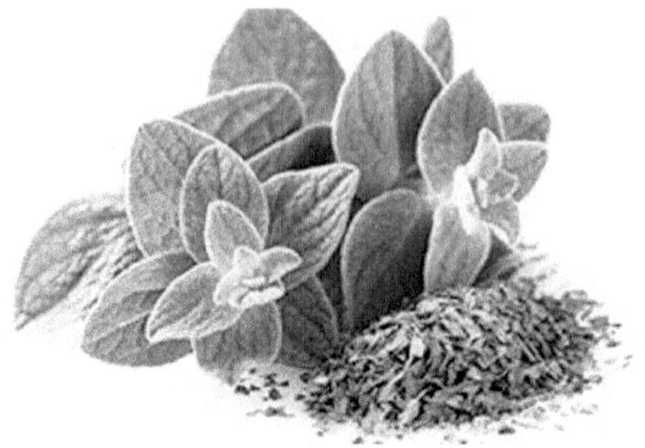

It is suitable for Italian food and tomato-based food items like pasta, pizza, and soups. It can be sprinkled on cheeses sandwiches or as an extra topping.

Rosemary

It is proven to aid in reducing inflammation in different parts of the body. Rosemary is believed to be highly beneficial for its effect on the heart and its health.

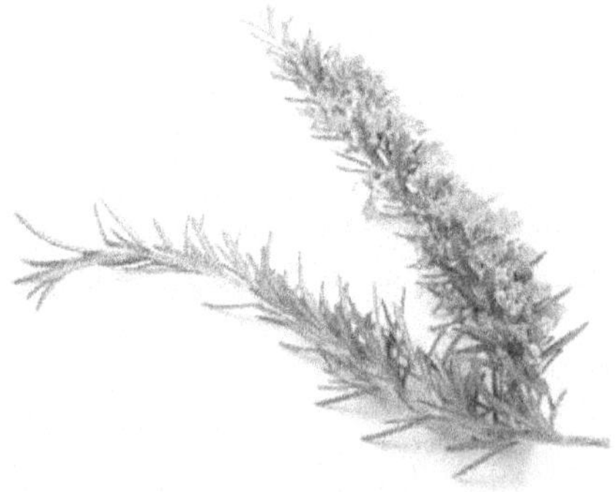

Rosemary can be added to marinades for sauces and meats. Various homemade wraps and bread receipts include rosemary both is crushed and raw form.

Turmeric

Turmeric is also included in the culinary herb group and is believed to lessen inflammation. The role of turmeric in detoxification of liver is also prominent. It is also being researched for the curative benefits for brain health.

As these are helpful in enhancing brain function so it prevents the decline of brain cells which usually occurs because of aging. Turmeric is used mostly in Asia where it is used as curry powder. It is also used after stirring curry powder into salad, egg salad, chicken salad, or even in tuna salad.

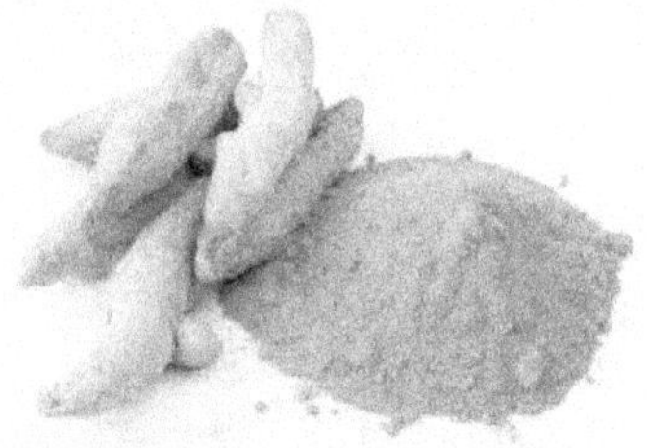

Cayenne

It is believed to help in various gastric issues and stomach problems. Cayenne is also helpful for   intestine function and increases the rate of metabolism which aids in weight control. It also soothes a sore throat, flu, and cold symptoms.

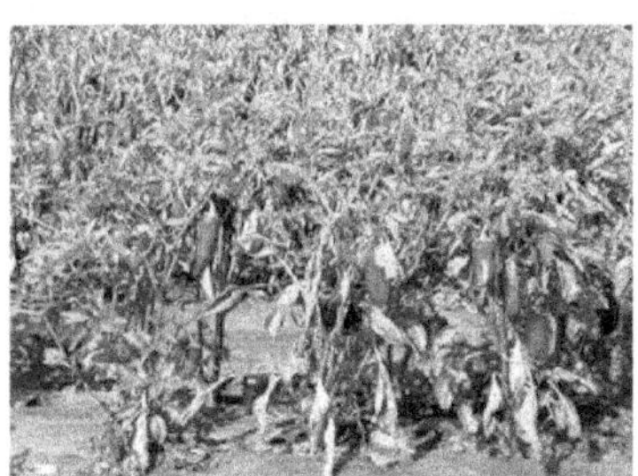

Chapter 3 – Tips to Grow, Dry, and Preserve Medicinal Herbs

Just as the exploration and research regarding medicines and the therapeutic phenomenon are increasing, there has been a rise in the use of botanic and herbal medicine.

As a result, there has been an extensive variety of ready to use natural and herbal remedies which have made their place onto the multiple shelves of herb stores, suppliers and at various chemists. These remedies are showing their effects so household customers are gaining interest in these herbs.

Although medicinal herbs are variable at the chemist and suppliers yet household customers are gaining interest to have these useful herbs at their home so that an enhanced level of effectiveness and utility can be achieved.

Growing herbs are easy yet it demands knowledge and some useful points for consideration. Below are some tips which can help in attaining greater production of herbs.

Collection of suitable Medicinal herbs

The first step for the effective growth of herbs is to gain knowledge about the availability of medicinal herb in the particular geographical region. Not all plants are suitable to be grown in all types of geographical location.

Although some artificial arrangements can be made yet if you are growing the herbs at the household level so arranging for these artificial conditions may turn out to be costly. You can also consult your nearest center of agriculture in order to gain proper guidance about the kind of medicinal herbs which can be grown in that area.

Identify the particular species☐

Even a single herb may have different species so the biggest challenge is to identify the correct species of the herb which is proven to have the medicinal benefits. Some herbs are nearly same in appearance with the sibling species. Apart from physical properties the chemical properties also matter so it is important to consult the herbal authorities in the locality.

Never grow across the Highway

Some herbs such as the Blackberry, Raspberry, and Ground Ivy have an inquisitive attraction for the lead which is given away by the fumes of the car-exhaust. So it is better to grow all the herbs after one mile from the highway. It will reduce the capacity of the herbal plant to reduce lead and hence the natural capacities of herbs will remain high.

Take the herb from correct Area

When you are ready to start your garden for herbs it is advisable to get the herb seedling from an area where the herb growth is highest so that your seedling can give you the highest growth. A seedling taken from a compromised place will, in turn, affect the eventual growth of herbs in your garden.

Harvest in the appropriate season

When growing herbs the most important thing is to consider the particular season which is considered to be most appropriate for the growth of the plant.

This information is readily available at the supplier store and other agriculture authorities. If harvested in the wrong season, a herb can never give an eventual growth and hence the growth will be compromised.

Tips for storing

- Heat, light, and air can cause the loss of taste and effectiveness in dried herbs. Moreover, the aroma may not remain same so it is better to keep them away from light and heat. ☐

- Store the dried herbs, bath medicinal as well culinary, in air-tight containers with fixed lids.

- a cupboard with a lock or a drawer will be the most suitable place to store herbs

- Do not keep the jars of the herbs above any appliance which is believed to produce heat such as dishwasher, microwave oven or refrigerator.

- While using the dried herbs do not sprinkle it from the jar as the jar may get moisture of the cooking pan which may damage the aroma and effectiveness of the remaining herbs.

- You can store the herbs for 1 year if these are in the form of ground spices or herbs and spices. For raw or whole herbs the storage time can be as long as two years.

- Label each of the containers with appropriate tag mentioning the date of preservation and name of the herb. It will ensure a safe usage.

•

Chapter 4 – How to Grow, Dry and Preserve Medicinal Herbs

Medicinal herbs, because of their intimate benefits are under discussion at the household level and people are interested in growing these herbs at home.

Below mentioned details provide an account of all the major aspects related to growth and preservation of medicinal herb. Follow these guidelines in the correct way in order to attain the maximum benefit out of these herbs.

Cultivation

Growing herbs is obviously a tedious task in which you will need to keep an eye on a number of related aspects.

- **Evaluate the climatic features**

The foremost point in growing medicinal herbs is to recognize the particular characteristics of the geographical zone so that the appropriate herb can be selected accordingly.

The geographical location put the important effect on growing herbs but these are not the sole sources. Within a larger climatic zone small "microclimates" can be arranged within the protected locations but these require extra arrangements and care.

- **Test the soil**

The soil is the potential source which serves as the hub of all those nutrients which are needed for plant growth. So the quality of soil will affect the success of the growth of a particular herb which you want to grow. A vast majority of the herbs grown in the

Mediterranean region are most of the time under sunny conditions. It is because these herbs need gritty soil along with excellent drainage. Another crucial factor to be determined is the pH factor. If the soil is having too acidic or too alkaline pH factor it can restrict the availability of all those nutrients which are vital for herb growth.

Drainage is also a crucial factor in determining before selecting the herb to be cultivated. A restricted drainage will hinder growth just like a quick drainage which moves away the nutrients too quickly.

You can test the drainage of the soil by applying following major steps:

Dig up a hole in the special area at which you want to grow the hole. The hole must be of the size equal to the gallon jug.

Now add water in the hole and allow it to drain. When the water will drain out completely, fill the hole with water again.

Note the time of water which it looks for drainage. On average, the drainage time must not be more than 8 hours. If it is so then before growing the herb you need to improve the drainage of the area.

- **Make compost:**

Compost is used for the organic enrichment of the soil. As the ecological emphasis for recycling is enhanced day by day so you can utilize your kitchen and yard waste in order to make up the best compost for your herb garden. The local agricultural authorities can help you in providing the complete plans for making appropriate compost as per the need of particular herb species. ☐

- **Mulching**

A mulching layer made of 3 to 4 inches can lessen the requirement of weeding and cultivation. It will aid to lessen the moisture loss and thus decrease the frequent need of watering.

Mulch can be made of barks, wood chips, gravel, shredded newspapers, sand or compost. Make sure to leave an inch space near the crown part of the plant so that excessive moisture mat does not induce rot or disease. ☐

- **Fertilizing**

In the case of herbs, the need for fertilizing is minimal. Excess use of fertilizer enhances the growth of the leaves and this compromises the presence of volatile oils which add medicinal properties to the herbs. Try to use natural fertilizer so that the herbs remain in the purest form.

- **Watering**

The frequency of watering needed by a particular herb will not depend upon the individual requirements of the herb but on the particular soil and climate conditions as well. So determine all the factors so that appropriate watering frequency id ensured.

Garden herbs usually need around one inch of water in one week. However, if the leaves of the herb grow actively then the plant will need more moisture. Dormant herbs will need lesser moisture. If climatic conditions are dry and hot then frequent watering will be needed.

Herbs garden with a lot of sandy soil will need even more water as compared to the one having heavier soil. It is highly critical to determine the specific needs of a species because apart from the climatic conditions the nature of the species will matter. □

Staking

Staking is the additional support provided to the herb stems in order to make them stand erect. Staking is usually needed by the loose herbs. Insert the staking support while the herb is at an average height because when it will become taller, it will be hard to induce staking.

Various different sizes of stakes may be needed for a normal herb grown in your garden. You may need multiple stakes for a large plant. Each part of the plant will then be staked to a part of support.

Any of the loose herbs may need a stake and ring combination. Some Other beneficial cavalries are tiny branches and multiple sizes of a stem. The least noticeable method will be a metal ring having a grid placed inside and then supported with three stakes. You can get these staking arrangements from local garden stores. The plant then carries on its growth along with the grid, finally wrapping it fully.

- **Propagation of herbs**

Herbs usually propagate from cuttings, seeds, layering or division. Seeds may be propagated outdoors after the soil becomes warm, indoor seedling can also occur in a tray before six weeks of planting time. In this case artificially prepared mixture will be provided in the tray.

Making the appropriate garden design

- **Garden Plans**

The type and size of garden solely depend on upon personal need, space, time and family preference. It is more appropriate to start the garden with a modest number of plants which can be increased later on, once the experience and knowledge increases. A herb garden can be a bit informal, having a mixture of flowers, herbs, and vegetables. But you can also choose a formal garden plan having herbs and paths laid out in an appropriate pattern.

Paths along the garden can be made of various different materials, like brick, grass, gravel, stone, or wood chips. But in every case, the path of the garden must be wide enough to handle mower or garden cart. However, if you want to grow herbs at a limited scale then you can also make your garden plan in patio, walking area or balcony.

- **Garden Site**

Choose some appropriate area for the growth of herbs. The area must get sunlight at least six hours a day. In northern parts of the world, the strongest sunlight is attained during the afternoon. Likewise southern parts of world support herbs which get benefit from shades. So, in that case, you will need to choose some shady herbs.

- **Choosing the plant**

A herb may grow from a tree, vine, shrub or even bulb. However, most of the herbs usually appear to be non-woody in character and hence named as herbaceous. A number of herbs like lavender, hyssop and rosemary may appear as semi-shrubs having woody stems. The annual herbs grow once in a year and biennials have two seasons in which leaves are to be produced first followed by the growth of a flower. So choose the plant appropriately

Collect the garden tools

A successful herb garden largely depends on upon the availability and use of the right tools. Select tools which are strong and long-lasting so that they can serve you for long.

For an average sized herb garden you will need spade, rake, spading fork trowel, cultivator, pruning shears, watering can, scissors, raffia or Tape, a hose and plant stakes. If you cannot get all of these then the least you will need will be the sturdy trowel, pruning shears, spade and a watering can.

Garden maintenance

An appropriate plan for garden maintenance will comprise of:

- Pruning and harvesting

- Garden clean up

- Winter protection

All these steps will eventually yield a good quantity of medicinal and eatable herbs for your use.

Drying of herbs

One of the most important parts comes when you have to dry the herbs. Again you need to be knowledgeable enough to choose the best drying technique for the particular herb in hand.

- Air drying

- Microwave drying

- Indoor drying

- Drying with the help of desiccants

- Drying in place

These are the various techniques of drying which can be chosen based on particular type of herb. Some species of herbs are quite easy to dry. The ones having strong leaves are a bit difficult to dry.

Although it is better to know it beforehand but trial and error will eventually make you learn about the appropriate type of drying technique. Some herbs will turn into brown messy texture after getting dried while others may not change their texture and color. The easiest to dry herbs include bay leaves, thyme, rosemary, and sage.□

Preserving the herbs

Preserving the herbs is necessary in order to increase the utility of the herbs, after the application of some suitable preservation technique the herbs can be utilized for more than a year. Some of the most common herb preserving technique is:

- Hanging

- Freezing

- Use of oil□

- Using paper towel

- Dehydrating

After applying the suitable preservation technique it is better to keep them in air tight jars at a dark place so that the direct sunlight may not change the flavor and taste.

Although growing herbs is an important task yet preserving these herbs is equally important. If you want to increase the storage life of these herbs you need to follow the important tips and procedures which are usually involved in storing herbs. Herbs can give you maximum benefit only when you are equipped with suitable knowledge.

Chapter 5 – Recipes to Use Medicinal and Culinary Herbs

Below are some of the recipes which involve the use of multiple culinary and medicinal herbs in a number of ways.

Basil Pesto

Ingredients:

- Basil leaves - 3 cups

- Garlic peeled - 2 cloves

- Pine nuts – 2 tbsp

- Sunflower seeds – 1 tbsp

- Salt- 1/4 tsp.

- Olive oil - 1/2 cup

- Parmesan cheese- 1/4 cup

Directions:

Take an electric blender and add garlic along with salt. Blend for at least 30 seconds. Now add basil leaves and now use the pulse technique by turning on and off the blender very often. It will shred the leaves evenly. While the blender will be still on, add olive oil to form a coarse mash. Now mix the Parmesan

Cheese and pulse again to combine.it will approximately make 1cup for serving.

Pico de Gallo

Ingredients:

- Plum tomatoes- 4 ripe

- White onion – 1 small

- Fresh cilantro (chopped)- 1/2 cup

- 1-2 jalapenos – 1-2

- Lime juice- 1 tablespoon

- Salt – to taste

Directions:

Mix all of the ingredients to thoroughly combine. Cover the bowl and refrigerate for one hour before serving.

Ginger Veggie

Ingredients:

- Head broccoli - 1 small

- Carrots- 3/4 cup

- Green beans (halved) - 1/2 cup

- Onion (chopped) - 1/4 cup

- Snow peas - 1/2 cup

- Garlic - 2 cloves

- Ginger root (minced) - 2 tbsp

- Vegetable oil - 1/4 cup

- Cornstarch - 1 tablespoon

- Soy sauce – 1 tablespoon

- Water – 2 tbsp

Directions:

Take a large bowl to mix garlic, cornstarch, ginger and vegetable oil till cornstarch gets easily dissolved. Now Mix in broccoli, carrots, snow peas, and green Beans. Toss evenly to lightly coat. Take 2 tablespoons of oil in a spate skillet and heat at a low flame.

Add vegetables and cool for almost two minutes. Make sure to stir continually so that vegetables may not burn. Cook evenly. Add water and soy sauce and water. Now Mix in salt, onion, and ginger. Keep moving spatula in vegetables so that the vegetables remain tender. Now add chicken in this mixture to serve as a complete meal.

Dandelion and vinegar mixture:

This mixture will be a tangy one with refreshing vinegar syrup mixed with the aromatics strawberries and the mineral-rich content of the special dandelion root. Mix these dandelion roots in a drink to beat the heat of a hot summer day and quench your thirst. Dandelion has soothing effects on the nerves and overall body. □

Conclusion

One of the most remarkable features of nature is the ingrained utility in every living being. From the giant creations to the tiniest entity every living being served some purpose.

It is the intelligence and exploration put forward by the human mind which determines the ultimate utility confined within every being. The same stands true in the case of botanical species which constitute a wide range of useful and helpful creations used in one way or the other. The vast number of these species calls for an overwhelming research and exploration so that the eventual benefit of these botanical entities can be attained.

Among the botanical species, herbs are one of the most useful species having millions of useful elements within them. Just as medical and food industry is extending greater research efforts about these species, a number of utilities which were once unknown, are being unveiled. These natural herbs constitute an additional benefit as they are the purest and natural so the absence of any artificial additions makes them even more useful.

As the utility of these herbs is getting a wider canvas people are now interested in growing these herbs at the individual level. This book is aimed to guide all such herb lovers so that they can grow various medicinal and culinary herbs in their garden and attain self-sufficient herb store at their homes. The basic knowledge once attained can be polished with practical experience so start at a small level and expand it with every passing day and additional experience gained.

FREE Bonus Reminder

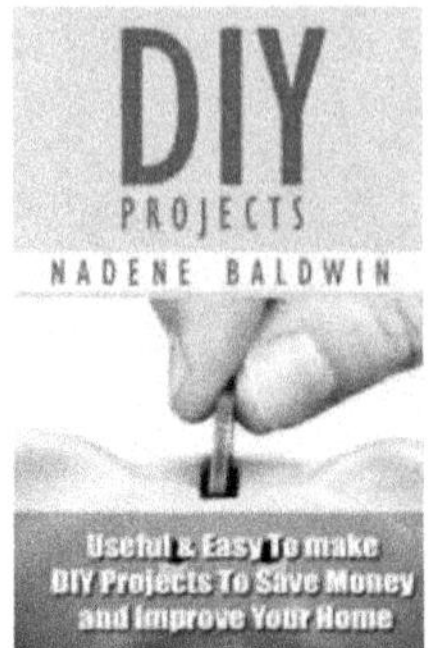

If you have not grabbed it yet, please go ahead and download your special bonus report *"DIY Projects. 13 Useful & Easy To Make DIY Projects To Save Money & Improve Your Home!"*

Simply Click the Button Below

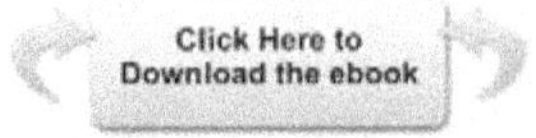

OR **Go to This Page**

http://diyhomecraft.com/free

BONUS #2: More Free & Discounted Books or Products

Do you want to receive more Free/Discounted Books or Products?

We have a mailing list where we send out our new Books or Products when they go free or with a discount on Amazon. Click on the link below to sign up for Free & Discount Book & Product Promotions.

=> Sign Up for Free & Discount Book & Product Promotions <=

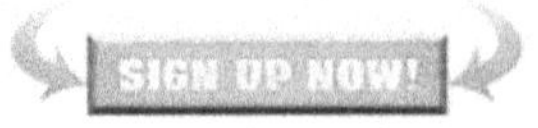

OR Go to this URL

http://zbit.ly/1WBb1Ek